Contents

Introduction

Over 6 million Americans suffer from fibromyalgia symptoms, and 90 percent of fibromyalgia sufferers are women. It's still up for debate why far more women get fibromyalgia than men. Some healthcare professionals claim it's due to decreased serotonin levels in the brains of women.

Unfortunately, people suffering from fibromyalgia struggle with pain, fatigue, depression and other common fibromyalgia symptoms prior to diagnosis.

Much like other chronic conditions, including adrenal fatigue, chronic fatigue syndrome and several rheumatoid conditions, there is not an immediate cure to relieve the often debilitating symptoms. In fact, these conditions share many of the same symptoms and, for some individuals, may occur in tandem.

Fibromyalgia is characterized by a phenomenon called central sensitization, in which pain receptors in the central nervous system (called nociceptors) become hyperreactive.3 This greatly amplifies sensitivity to pain and can be triggered by things like illness, infection, injury, stress, and, for some people, food.

A review Journal of Human Nutrition and Diet suggests food intolerance and hypersensitivity affects around half of all people living with fibromyalgia.

Fibromyalgia's relationship to food intolerance is unclear, but some scientists believe allergy plays a role. In one study in Clinical and Translational Science, no less than 49% of people with fibromyalgia had at least one food allergy, while 50% tested strongly positive for a milk allergy. Intolerance to wheat, another common food allergen, also occurred.

It is possible that a hypersensitive food reaction can trigger fibromyalgia symptoms as the body releases pro-inflammatory compounds, called cytokines, into the bloodstream. Cytokines not only help instigate food allergies but are linked to the onset of fibromyalgia symptoms, most especially hyperalgesia (increased pain sensitivity).

Other experts contend that any food intolerance can provoke fibromyalgia by triggering inflammation in the gut that can "spill over" to the nociceptors in the brain. These include common causes like gluten (associated with celiac disease and gluten intolerance) and FODMAPs (fermentable sugars linked to irritable bowel syndrome, or IBS).

Chapter one

Common Fibromyalgia Symptoms

The severity of fibromyalgia symptoms varies from person to person, and often, symptoms disappear and then return. Fibromyalgia is characterized by long-term and widespread pain in muscles and connective tissues, without any specific cause.

Research has shown that fibromyalgia may actually amplify pain by affecting the way the brain processes pain signals. In addition to pain, common fibromyalgia symptoms include:

- Fatigue
- Headaches
- Memory issues
- Sleep disorders
- Cramping in the lower abdomen
- Tender points
- Chronic pain
- Depression
- Anxiety
- Fibro fog

Are these symptoms of fibromyalgia chronic? In many cases, yes. And while the pain associated with fibromyalgia is challenging for many, "fibro fog" and sleep disorders add to this challenging diagnosis.

Sleep disorders are common and may include sleep apnea and restless legs syndrome. Not getting enough sleep contributes to diminished cognitive functioning, depression and anxiety.

In addition, some patients experience morning stiffness, numbness or tingling in the extremities, as well as a heightened sensitivity to loud noises, bright lights and temperature. Some patients also experience fibromyalgia with other co-existing conditions including TMJ (temporomandibular joint dysfunction), endometriosis, chronic fatigue syndrome, tension headaches and IBS (irritable bowel syndrome).

Meanwhile, fibromyalgia syndrome (FMS) is a form of fibromyalgia "where pain and stiffness occurs in muscles, tendons, and ligaments throughout the body, accompanied by other generalized symptoms such as fatigue, sleep disruption, mood disorder and cognitive difficulties." (3b)

Fibromyalgia symptoms

Causes of Fibromyalgia Symptoms

It can be difficult to be diagnosed with fibromyalgia, as there isn't a definitive laboratory test. While blood work and other tests may be ordered in order to rule out other conditions, doctors often rely on feedback they receive from the patient.

In general, patients must experience widespread pain or muscle aches that last for at least three months. A physical "tender point" examination may be conducted where the doctor presses 18 specific points to measure pain and tenderness. Tender points include neck, chest, arms, legs near the knee, at the waist and just below the buttocks.

Some fibromyalgia patients may actually suffer from neuropathy, as a study found that almost half of the patients suffered from small nerve fiber neuropathy. That is simply nerve pain that is caused by damage to the small nerves which carry pain and other signals from your skin to your brain. Therefore, neuropathic fibromyalgia may be more common than previously known.

While there is neither a definitive nor singular cause for fibromyalgia, it's been linked to the following:

- Genetics
- Allergies to chemicals
- Food sensitivities or allergies
- Viruses
- Hormonal imbalances
- Poor digestion
- Candida overgrowth
- Spinal misalignments
- Stress

- Neurotransmitter deficiencies
- Stress

PTSD

Risk factors for fibromyalgia include genetics, being female, and rheumatoid arthritis or lupus. For some individuals, symptoms begin after a significant psychological stress event, infection, surgery or other physical trauma. Others may have no evidence of a triggering event, and the fibromyalgia symptoms have just accumulated over time.

More recently, one 2017 study found that patients with fibromyalgia (FM) have brains with abnormal hypersensitivity, otherwise known as explosive synchronization (ES). Researchers from the University of Michigan and Pohang University of Science reported that the hypersensitivity fibromyalgia patients experience may be a result from the hypersensitive or hyperactive brain networks.

Researchers analyzed the resting state electroencephalogram (EEG) — the test that records electrical signals of the brain — of 10 female fibromyalgia patients to examine well-known ES conditions within functional brain networks. Then, researchers tested whether a brain network model with ES conditions reacted to external disturbances or electrical stimulation. From this research, external disturbances greatly correlate with chronic pain intensity, and the data supports that networks with ES conditions are more sensitive to disturbances compared to brains without ES networks. Furthermore, explosive synchronization may be a mechanism of fibromyalgia brain hypersensitivity, according to the findings of the study. The model of this test and research can assist future treatments of fibromyalgia that could potentially transform fibromyalgia hypersensitivity networks into stable networks using noninvasive brain modulation therapies.

Treating Fibromyalgia Symptoms

Traditional treatment for fibromyalgia includes nonsteroidal anti-inflammatory drugs (NSAIDS), anti-seizure drugs, pain relievers and antidepressants. Lyrica (pregabalin) is one of the most common FDA-approved drug treatments for fibromyalgia. These commonly prescribed fibromyalgia medications don't cure the disease, and taking them can cause potentially serious side effects.

NSAIDS can cause ulcers, bleeding in the stomach or intestines, digestive upset, high blood pressure, heart attack, stroke and even life-threatening skin reactions and allergic reactions. While inflammation is a problem, there are better natural alternatives.

Side effects of prescription anti-seizure medications include liver failure, kidney stones, ovarian cysts, along with serious drops in white blood cells and number of platelets, aplastic anemia and cognitive function problems.

Prescription antidepressants can cause weight gain, loss of sexual desire, fatigue, insomnia, blurred vision, agitation, irritability and anxiety. Several of these potential side effects are similar to common symptoms of fibromyalgia. Several supplements are available to help relieve depression and anxiety (see below).

Treating fibromyalgia symptoms naturally requires a healthy diet, changes in lifestyle and complementary treatments. Since fibromyalgia can cause chronic pain and fatigue that is similar to arthritis, some experts may advise a fibromyalgia patient to see a rheumatologist. While there isn't a cure yet, there are natural treatments that can help ease the symptoms and increase the quality of life for fibromyalgia sufferers.

Fibromyalgia Diet & Natural Treatment

Multiple clinical studies show that treating fibromyalgia symptoms requires a multi-pronged approach that includes changes in diet and nutrition. A collaborative study from researchers in Italy have found that fibromyalgia patients can benefit from specific dietary changes and nutritional supplementation.

This study found that the elimination of gluten has the potential for improving symptoms of fibromyalgia. This result is echoed in another recent study published in Arthritis Research & Therapy, where researchers studied the effect of a one-year gluten-free diet in patients with co-occurring IBS and fibromyalgia.

In fact, one of the subgroups in the study experienced significant improvement in all symptoms and an improvement in quality of life scores.

Of foods to avoid when treating fibromyalgia, gluten is obviously key. Researchers from both the studies above encourage more research and further study of recommended dietary and nutritional changes for fibromyalgia patients.

In addition to eliminating gluten, it's essential to limit caffeine intake, as it can contribute to restless sleep and insomnia, anxiety, muscle tremors and depression – many of the symptoms fibromyalgia patients experience everyday.

Remember, caffeine lurks not only in coffee, tea and colas but also in energy drinks, non-cola flavored sodas and even some over-the-counter pain medications. Currently, the FDA doesn't require caffeine to be listed on nutrition labels. This makes it difficult for individuals trying to limit or avoid caffeine.

Be mindful of chocolate bars, as some manufacturers add caffeine to their recipe, as well as diet pills and some deceptive processed foods marketed as "perky" or "morning spark."

I recommend to all my patients to avoid artificial sweeteners at all costs. Made from dangerous chemicals, many common artificial sweeteners on the market today contain compounds linked to cancer, thyroid conditions, memory loss and seizures.

When fighting the symptoms of fibromyalgia, it's important to not stimulate further complications and medical conditions. Reducing your body's toxic burden by eliminating gluten, caffeine, artificial sweeteners, processed foods and partially hydrogenated oils and trans fats, you can make a difference in how you feel and in your quality of life.

Foods to Include in a Fibromyalgia Diet

Now let's look at a healthy fibromyalgia diet. Replace the foods mentioned above with nutrient-dense clean proteins, raw dairy, fermented foods, organic fruits and vegetables and other foods listed in my healing foods diet.

Many fibromyalgia patients have underlying nutritional deficiencies and may be deficient in key nutrients including vitamins B12, C, and D, as well as folic acid and the essential mineral magnesium. The goal is to reduce inflammation and build the body's natural defenses. Simply put, this requires a change in diet, a radical change for some people.

Magnesium-Rich Foods: Include lots of green leafy vegetables, pumpkin seeds, yogurt or kefir, almonds, and avocados in your diet to increase magnesium levels. Aim for a minimum of three servings a day of these foods to help ease the pain and discomfort associated with fibromyalgia.

Melatonin-Rich Foods: As sleep disorders are common among fibromyalgia symptoms, increasing the sleep hormone melatonin is recommended. Melatonin supplements are considered generally safe, but it can interact with certain medications, including immunosuppressants, birth control pills, anticoagulants and diabetic prescriptions.

Fortunately, there are many foods you can eat to get the melatonin you need! Melatonin-rich foods include the following:

- Tart/Sour Cherries and Cherry Juice
- Walnuts
- Mustard Seed
- Rice
- Ginger
- Barley
- Asparagus
- Tomatoes
- Fresh Mint
- Bananas
- Red Wine

Studies show that deficiencies in zinc, magnesium and folate are linked with lower melatonin levels. This is why it's essential on a fibromyalgia diet to eat foods rich in essential nutrients.

Foods High in Tryptophan: Tryptophan is needed by the body to produce serotonin, which is associated with restful sleep. When people think of tryptophan, they often think of turkey but there are other healthy foods with high tryptophan levels — including nuts, grass-fed dairy, wild fish, free-range chicken, sprouted grain, and sesame seeds — that can help you sleep.

Coconut Oil: Replace all unhealthy fats with coconut oil. Incorporate three to four tablespoons per day into your diet to help reduce joint pain, balance hormones, improve memory and overall brain function.

Fermented Foods and Drinks: Kombucha and other fermented products help to restore a healthy floral balance to the gut. As many sufferers of fibromyalgia also have IBS, it's important to improve digestion. Sauerkraut and kefir should also be incorporated to the fibromyalgia diet to help relieve 'fibro fog,' aches and pains.

Wild Fish: Salmon and tuna are excellent sources of omega-3 fatty acids and other essential vitamins and minerals. For people with fibromyalgia and other rheumatoid conditions, wild fish and fish oil are essential. In fact, omega-3 supplements can curb stiffness, joint pain, lower depression and improve mental skills.

Turmeric: Add freshly grated turmeric (or curcumin) to your favorite recipes. Curcumin is the active ingredient renowned for its antioxidant and anti-inflammatory effects. To help the body absorb it properly, it's important to consume turmeric with black pepper.

Ginger: This proven strong anti-inflammatory spice helps to relieve pain. In a randomized, double-blind, placebo-controlled study in Miami, researchers found study participants given ginger experienced a greater reduction in knee pain than those given acetaminophen.

The group receiving the ginger extract did experience more stomach upset than those receiving the acetaminophen, although digestive upset was mild. Add fresh ginger to salad dressings, marinades and other favorite recipes.

Goals of a Fibromyalgia Diet

An individualized fibromyalgia diet aims to:

Identify food intolerances and sensitivities so foods that cause gastrointestinal symptoms and trigger fibromyalgia flares can be avoided:

Avoid foods and additives known to stimulate nociceptors in the brain. These include those high in an amino acid known as glutamate. Glutamate functions as a neurotransmitter and is found in abnormally high concentrations in the brains of people with fibromyalgia.[6]

Compensate for nutritional deficiencies common in people with fibromyalgia. These include deficiencies in iron, iodine, magnesium, selenium, vitamin D, and vitamin B12.[7]

Planning Your Fibromyalgia Diet

Although some specialists will recommend specific diets for people with fibromyalgia, there is no set group of foods that affects all people in the same way.

For that reason, developing a fibromyalgia diet plan starts with the process of identifying the foods you are sensitive to and the ones you can eat safely. It may also involve eating more foods that are high in magnesium, selenium, vitamin D, and vitamin B12 to maintain control over hyperalgesia.

Fibromyalgia Elimination Diet

An effective way to figure out which foods are troublesome is with the type of elimination diet used to diagnose things like IBS, food allergies, and gluten sensitivity.

To do an elimination diet, it's best to work with a healthcare provider or dietitian to prevent malnutrition or nutritional deficiencies that could lead to new problems as you follow these steps:8

Make a list of the foods (for example, eggs or nuts) or food groups (dairy, grains, etc.) you suspect may be causing problems.

Avoid everything on the list for two weeks. Do not eat these foods whole or as an ingredient in a prepared dish.

If your symptoms don't improve after two weeks, your healthcare provider or nutritionist may advise you to stop the diet and consider other possible food and non-food triggers.

If fibromyalgia symptoms resolve after two weeks, introduce one food group back into the diet every three days.

On the day a food is reintroduced, eat a small amount in the morning. If you don't have symptoms, eat two larger portions in the afternoon and evening. You should then stop eating the food for two days to see if you develop any symptoms. If you don't, the food is unlikely to be a trigger.

If a food is reintroduced and triggers symptoms, make note of it in a diary and tell your healthcare provider. Wait another two days before re-challenging yourself with another food group on the list.

Cooking Tips

A fibromyalgia diet focuses largely on whole foods prepared simply. Frying or deep-frying should be avoided and replaced with grilling, broiling, or steaming. If you decide to pan-fry, use a spray bottle to add as little oil as possible to the pan (ideally extra virgin olive oil).

Some studies suggest that the less you cook your food, the better. This includes research suggesting that a raw vegetarian diet may reduce hyperalgesia in some people with fibromyalgia.

- Prepare Ahead for Success

A common challenge with trying to follow an elimination diet like this is having healthy food at the ready. If you don't have a lot of time to cook during the work week, consider prepping ahead of time. Make several fibromyalgia-friendly meals in advance, and freeze in individual serving sizes. That way you will be able to stick to your eating plan when short on time.

- Choosing a Fibromyalgia Diet Plan to Follow

Many experts recommend choosing a Mediterranean diet to follow both because of how healthy it is and how sustainable it is to follow over the long term. US News ranked it as the number 1 diet.

There is lots of evidence to suggest a Mediterranean-style diet can help with the following:

- Protect against type 2 diabetes
- Reduce inflammation

- Reduce the risk of heart disease, stroke, and diabetes
- Reduce weight sustainably
- The main characteristics of eating a Mediterranean diet are typical of a balanced diet and include:
- High unsaturated-to-saturated fat ratio
- High consumption of fruits, vegetables, legumes, nuts and unrefined grains
- Increased consumption of fish
- Moderate consumption of low-fat dairy (mostly cheese and yogurt)
- Limited intake of red meat and processed foods

Various credible organizations recommend following a Mediterranean diet to help with diabetes, including:

- Harvard Medical School
- Mayo Clinic
- American Heart Association
- Arthritis Foundation
- Fibromyalgia Diet Meal Plan
- Sample Menu

In the meal plan are recipes for breakfast, lunch and dinner.

Breakfast Lunch Dinner

Mon Blueberry Blues Porridge Greek Salad Haddock Risotto

Tues Basil & Spinach Scramble Falafel Wraps Eggplant & Lentil Bake

Wed Tomato & Watermelon Salad Carrot, Orange & Avocado Salad Mediterranean Chicken, Quinoa & Greek Salad

Thurs Blueberry Blues Porridge Mixed Bean Salad Grilled Vegetables with Bean Mash

Fri Basil & Spinach Scramble Panzanella Salad Salmon & Chickpea Salad

Sat Tomato & Watermelon Salad Spiced Carrot & Lentil Soup Chicken Gyros

Sun Blueberry Blues Porridge Moroccan Chickpea Soup Spicy Mediterranean Beet Salad

Snacks are recommended between meal times. Some good snacks include:

- A handful of nuts or seeds
- A piece of fruit
- Carrots or baby carrots
- Berries or grapes

A healthy diet, lifestyle changes and nutritional supplements are all part of the equation for fighting the symptoms of fibromyalgia.

Here are today's best supplements for battling fibromyalgia:

Acetyl L-carnitine (1500 mg/day): A small randomized trial tested acetyl L-carnitine and prescription duloxetine (Cymbalta) in 65 women with fibromyalgia. While both led to a general clinical improvement, the study found that the acetyl L-carnitine may improve depression, pain and the overall quality of life in fibromyalgia patients.

Magnesium (500 mg/day): As mentioned above, magnesium deficiency is often linked to fibromyalgia. Increasing magnesium can help to reduce pain and tenderness. In addition, it helps to increase energy and reduce both anxiety and depression.

Fish Oil (1000 mg/day): Fish oil supplements replace omega-6 fatty acids in the brain with healthy omega-3s. (22) Fish oil is one of nature's richest sources of omega-3 fatty acids and can help relieve anxiety, depression and improve brain function.

Turmeric & Black Pepper Combo (1000 mg/day): As mentioned above, it's important to take it with black pepper. Fortunately, there are high-quality combination supplements available. A study recently published in Clinical Nutrition found supplements containing curcuminoids and piperine significantly improves inflammation and oxidative status.

Vitamin D3 (5,000 IU/day): A deficiency in vitamin D is associated with chronic pain in some individuals. One small study found the control group that received the vitamin D supplementation experienced a marked reduction in pain. Researchers believe larger studies are warranted.

Rhodiola and Ashwagandha (500-1000 mg/day); Anxiety, exhaustion, stress and hormone imbalances are common in fibromyalgia patients. Together, these two adaptogens work together to help the body effectively respond to stress.

5-Hydroxytryptophan/5-HTP (50 mg 1-3 times/day): 5-HTP may help to increase deep sleep, while relieving pain. It works by supporting healthy serotonin levels in the brain. It's made in the body from tryptophan, but is not found in foods high in tryptophan. Supplementation is necessary.

According to a small placebo-controlled study for fibromyalgia and 5-HTP, symptoms of fibromyalgia can be improved with supplements. Supplements of 5-HTP are made from the Griffonia simplicifolia seeds and are safe for most individuals.

Lifestyle Changes for Fibromyalgia

The potential for lifestyle changes to help fibromyalgia symptoms cannot be glossed over. Nonmedical intervention is necessary to relieve symptoms, including a healthy fibromyalgia diet and supplements. Chiropractic care, reducing stress, regular exercise, acupuncture and massage therapy can all be helpful.

Regular Moderate Exercise: For many people in the midst of a fibromyalgia flare, the last thing that sounds appealing is exercise. That is understandable considering the pain and exhaustion. However, regular moderate exercise that includes walking, swimming, biking, yoga and Pilates can help relieve stress and pain.

A study published in the Archives of Physical Medicine & Rehabilitation found a strong relationship between physical fitness and fibromyalgia. Higher physical fitness levels are consistently associated with less severe symptoms in women.

Yoga: An eight-week study considering the benefits of yoga in pain relief found that 75-minute yoga sessions, twice per week, reduces pain. In addition, it altered total cortisol levels in women with fibromyalgia and increased mindfulness.

Acupuncture: For over 2,500 years, acupuncture has been used to relieve pain, increase relaxation and so much more. A small study has found that acupuncture is a proven, safe and effective treatment for the immediate reduction of pain in patients with fibromyalgia.

Researchers believe that acupuncture works by restoring normal balance in the body and pain relief comes from the opioid peptides released during the session. Many believe this is the body's natural response for managing pain. When systems are off-balance and energy isn't flowing properly, acupuncture can help.

Massage Therapy: Regular massage reduces heart rate, relieves pain, improves range of motion, and lessens anxiety and depression. Weekly massages are recommended for continued relief.

Manual Lymph Drainage Therapy: A small study published in the Journal of Manipulative & Physiological Therapeutics found that MLDT helps moves lymph fluid through the body eliminating toxins and waste in fibromyalgia patients.

Clearing the body of toxins helps to stimulate healing and can relieve many of the symptoms associated with fibromyalgia.

Essential Oils: Essential oils are effective for treating a wide array of conditions and symptoms, including relieving stress and reducing pain. Helicrysum oil is shown to improve circulation, support the healing of nerve tissue and decrease muscle pain. Combine with coconut oil and massage into sore areas.

Lavender oil is known to help relieve emotional stress, improve sleep and reduce anxiety. Use in a homemade muscle rub to relieve pain and in a diffuser in the bedroom to help improve the quality of sleep.

Moist Heat: Moist heat boosts the blood flow to areas of the body in pain, providing relief. Warm baths (with a few drops of essential oils), showers and moist heating pads can help when in pain.

Get Some Sun(!): Aim for a minimum of 10-20 minutes of sunshine each day to naturally increase vitamin D levels. It's important during the sun exposure to not wear sunscreen, as it can prohibit the rays of sunshine you need.

The big challenge in fibromyalgia treatment is keeping hope alive. Researchers are striving to find the answers needed to treat this debilitating condition. Many of the world's leading researchers are considering natural fibromyalgia treatments; we have highlighted many of them here.

Consistently, healthcare professionals across the globe recommend complementary treatments that include diet, lifestyle changes and natural supplements. Continue to read about it at the National Institute of Arthritis and Musculoskeletal and Skin Diseases (NIAMS). The key is to find the right combination of these elements that works to help you relieve your fibromyalgia symptoms.

Chapter two

Fibromyalgia Diet Recipes

Koula's Best Ever Chicken Gyros

This is an unusual version of classic Middle Eastern gyros (only homemade under the oven's broiler). Very tasty and quick to make. Perfect weekday dinner! You can prepare it in advance, let it marinate and just stick it in the oven. Best served inside pita bread pockets, with salad and yogurt.

Prep Time: 10 mins

Cook Time: 20 mins

Total Time: 30 mins

Servings: 4

Yield: 4 servings

Ingredients

3 skinless, boneless chicken breast halves - cut into 1/2 inch strips

2 tablespoons ketchup

2 tablespoons olive oil

1 ½ teaspoons white wine vinegar

1 teaspoon dried oregano

1 teaspoon mustard powder

1 ½ teaspoons curry powder, or to taste

4 pita breads, cut in half

2 cups mixed salad greens

1 cup plain yogurt

Directions

Place the chicken strips side by side in a broiling pan. In a cup or small bowl, stir together the ketchup, olive oil, white wine vinegar, oregano, mustard powder and curry powder. Pour over the chicken. Allow the chicken to marinate while you preheat the oven's broiler.

Broil uncovered for 15 minutes with the meat about 6 inches from the heat. Just until the chicken is cooked through, but not browned. If left too long, it will turn stringy and dry.

Place hot chicken into pita pockets and spoon some of the juices from the pan over it. Top with salad greens and plain yogurt.

Nutrition Facts (per serving)

381 Calories 11g Fat 41g Carbs 28g Protein

Easy Chicken Gyro

Easy chicken gyro recipe with marinated chicken, fresh veggies, and homemade tzatziki on a warm pita round.

Prep Time: 30 mins

Cook Time: 20 mins

Additional Time: 1 hr

Total Time: 1 hr 50 mins

Servings: 6

Ingredients

Tzatziki:

1 (16 ounce) container Greek yogurt

1 medium cucumber, peeled and coarsely chopped

2 cloves garlic, minced

1 tablespoon extra-virgin olive oil

1 ½ teaspoons dried dill weed

1 teaspoon distilled white vinegar

1 teaspoon lemon juice

salt and ground black pepper to taste

Chicken:

4 cloves garlic, minced

1 medium lemon, juiced

2 tablespoons extra-virgin olive oil

1 tablespoon dried oregano

2 teaspoons red wine vinegar

salt and ground black pepper to taste

1 ¼ pounds skinless, boneless chicken breast halves - cut into strips

Gyros:

6 (6 inch) pita bread rounds

1 medium tomato, diced

1 medium red onion, thinly sliced

½ head iceberg lettuce, chopped

Directions

Gather all ingredients.

Make the tzatziki: Combine yogurt, cucumber, garlic, oil, dill, vinegar, lemon juice, salt, and pepper in a blender. Blend until smooth, then cover and refrigerate until needed.

Make the chicken: Whisk garlic, lemon juice, oil, oregano, vinegar, salt, and pepper together in a large glass or ceramic bowl. Add chicken and toss until evenly coated. Cover with plastic wrap and marinate in the refrigerator for 1 hour.

Preheat the oven's broiler and set the oven rack about 6 inches from the heat source. Line a rimmed baking sheet with foil.

Remove chicken from the marinade and place onto the prepared baking sheet.

Broil in the preheated oven until lightly browned and no longer pink in the center, 2 to 4 minutes per side. Transfer cooked chicken to a plate and let rest for 5 minutes.

While the chicken is resting, make the gyros: Heat a large nonstick skillet over medium heat. Cook each pita in the hot skillet until warm and soft, about 1 minute per side.

Top warm pitas with chicken strips, tzatziki, lettuce, tomato, and onion.

Enjoy!

Nutrition Facts (per serving)

441 Calories 18g Fat 39g Carbs 30g Protein

Vegetarian Moroccan Harira

Harira is a famous Moroccan soup, and here's a hearty vegetarian (and vegan!) version - packed with tomatoes and chickpeas and flavored with paprika, turmeric, saffron, ginger, and harissa. The amount of water can be adjusted depending on the thickness you want. I like this soup pretty thick and nourishing, so I do not add too much water.

Prep Time: 20 mins

Cook Time: 45 mins

Total Time: 1 hr 5 mins

Servings: 5

Yield: 5 servings

Ingredients

2 tablespoons vegetable oil

1 large onion, chopped

2 pounds tomatoes, diced

1 (15 ounce) can chickpeas, drained

1 bunch fresh cilantro, chopped

1 bunch fresh parsley, chopped

20 fresh mint leaves, chopped

1 teaspoon ground paprika

1 teaspoon ground turmeric

1 teaspoon ground ginger

½ teaspoon harissa

1 pinch saffron threads

4 cups water, or more to taste

1 tablespoon all-purpose flour

1 teaspoon cornstarch

½ cup cherry tomatoes, halved

salt and ground black pepper to taste

Directions

Heat oil in a large pot over medium heat and cook onion until soft and translucent, about 5 minutes. Add tomatoes, chickpeas, cilantro, parsley, mint, paprika, turmeric, ginger, harissa, and saffron. Add water and cook over medium heat until flavors have combined, about 30 minutes.

Mix a few tablespoons of soup liquid with flour and cornstarch in a small bowl and return to the soup, stirring in well. Add cherry tomatoes. Bring to a boil, reduce heat, and simmer over low heat until soup thickens, about 10 minutes. Season with salt and pepper.

Cook's Note:

If you have time, peel your tomatoes. To do this, cut an X on the bottom of each, submerge in boiling water for 25 seconds, transfer to an ice water bath, then peel gently and dice.

Nutrition Facts (per serving)

182 Calories

7g Fat

27g Carbs

6g Protein

Harira is Morocco's most popular soup. It is without a doubt one of the best soups you'll ever enjoy, and I am very happy to show you my take on this dish. Once you taste it you'll understand why the combination of pasta, lentils, and chickpeas is so hearty, so flavorful, and so satisfying. If you prefer a vegetarian harira soup, you can leave out the lamb.

Prep Time: 20 mins

Cook Time: 1 hr 20 mins

Total Time: 1 hr 40 mins

Servings: 6

Ingredients

2 tablespoons extra-virgin olive oil, plus more for garnish

12 ounces boneless lamb shoulder, cut into 1/2 -inch pieces (Optional)

1 large yellow onion, diced

1 teaspoon kosher salt, divided, or to taste

1 ½ teaspoons smoked paprika

1 teaspoon ground coriander

1 teaspoon ground cumin

½ teaspoon ground ginger

½ teaspoon freshly ground black pepper

¼ teaspoon ground cinnamon

4 cloves garlic, minced

1 tablespoon tomato paste

4 cups chicken broth

1 (15 ounce) can crushed tomatoes

2 ribs celery with leaves, chopped

2 cups water, or to taste

1 (15 ounce) can chickpeas, drained

¾ cup green lentils, rinsed

1 tablespoon all-purpose flour

2 tablespoons cold water

½ cup chopped fresh cilantro, divided

½ cup chopped fresh parsley, divided

½ cup vermicelli, broken into 1/2-inch pieces

⅛ teaspoon cayenne pepper

1 lemon, juiced

Directions

Gather all ingredients.

Heat olive oil in a stock pot over medium-high heat and cook cubed lamb until nicely browned and some of the fat has rendered, about 5 minutes.

Toss in diced onion and a generous pinch of salt. Cook, stirring often, until onion is soft and lightly browned, 4 to 5 minutes. Season with smoked paprika, coriander, cumin, ground ginger, black pepper, and cinnamon. Add minced garlic and cook and stir until fragrant, 30 seconds to 1 minute.

Add tomato paste and cook and stir for about 1 minute.

Add chicken broth, crushed tomatoes, and celery; stir until well combined. Add water and bring to a boil over high heat.

Once soup is boiling, add chickpeas and green lentils; season with salt to taste. Reduce heat to medium-low and simmer for 30 minutes, stirring occasionally.

Mix flour and 2 tablespoons cold water in a small bowl and drizzle slurry into the soup to thicken.

Bring back to a simmer and add 1/2 of the cilantro and 1/2 of the parsley; stir to combine.

Simmer on medium-low heat until meat and lentils are perfectly tender and soup has thickened, about 20 more minutes.

Stir in vermicelli and cook until tender, 10 to 15 minutes. Taste and adjust seasoning with cayenne and salt. Add remaining chopped cilantro and parsley and finish by drizzling lemon juice to taste into the soup.

Serve immediately with a drizzle of olive oil.

Nutrition Facts (per serving)

214 Calories 6g Fat 33g Carbs 10g Protein

Greek Salad

This Greek salad recipe is incredibly good! It's nice and tangy and tastes even better in the summer when tomatoes and cucumbers are at their best.

Prep Time: 20 mins

Total Time: 20 mins

Servings: 6

Can You Make Greek Salad Ahead of Time?

You can make the Greek salad dressing a few days in advance — just store it in the refrigerator until you're ready to use it. We recommend throwing the salad ingredients just before serving for the most delicious results.

Ingredients

1 head romaine lettuce- rinsed, dried and chopped

1 cucumber, sliced

2 large tomatoes, chopped

1 (6 ounce) can pitted black olives

1 green bell pepper, chopped

1 red bell pepper, chopped

1 red onion, thinly sliced

1 cup crumbled feta cheese

6 tablespoons olive oil

1 lemon, juiced

1 teaspoon dried oregano

ground black pepper to taste

Directions

Combine romaine, cucumber, tomatoes, olives, bell peppers, and red onion in a large bowl; sprinkle with feta cheese.

Whisk olive oil, lemon juice, oregano, and black pepper together in a small bowl. Pour dressing over salad, toss well to combine, and serve.

Pour dressing over salad, toss well to combine, and serve.

Nutrition Facts (per serving)

265 Calories 22g Fat 14g Carbs 6g Protein

This Greek salad dressing is the "secret recipe" from the pizzeria that I work at. This is the best dressing I have ever tasted, people offer to buy it constantly, but if we sold it we wouldn't be able to make enough to use in the restaurant! The recipe makes almost a gallon but can be scaled down easily.

Prep Time: 10 mins

Total Time 10 mins

Servings: 120

Yield: 1 gallon

How to Store Greek Dressing

This Greek dressing can be stored at room temperature (in an airtight container) if you plan to use it within a day or two. If you'd like to keep it for up to a week, you should store it in the refrigerator.

Ingredients

1 ½ quarts olive oil

⅓ cup garlic powder

⅓ cup dried oregano

⅓ cup dried basil

¼ cup ground black pepper

¼ cup salt

¼ cup onion powder

¼ cup Dijon-style mustard

2 quarts red wine vinegar

Directions

Gather all ingredients.

Mix olive oil, garlic powder, oregano, basil, pepper, salt, onion powder, and Dijon-style mustard together in a very large container. Pour in vinegar slowly while mixing vigorously until well blended. Store tightly covered at room temperature.

Pour over salad and enjoy!

Recipe Tip

This dressing is great for picnics and travels very well since it doesn't need to be refrigerated.

Nutrition Facts (per serving)

104 Calories 11g Fat 2g Carbs 0g Protein

You can't go wrong with this traditional Greek salad, especially if you remember the only and most important tip: toss it with the vinegar first before adding olive oil. If you don't, it will not taste as good. Which reminds me, giving the amounts here is very difficult, since this really should be made to your tastes, so please use the ingredient list as a very rough outline.

Prep Time: 20 mins

Additional Time: 50 mins

Total Time: 1 hr 10 mins

Servings: 4

Yield: 4

Ingredients

2 large English cucumbers

1 pinch kosher salt

2 cups cherry tomatoes

¼ red onion

½ red bell pepper

½ cup pitted Kalamata olives

½ cup pitted green olives

2 tablespoons minced fresh oregano

salt and freshly ground black pepper to taste

1 pinch cayenne pepper, or to taste

¼ cup red wine vinegar, or to taste

⅓ cup olive oil, or to taste

1 (4 ounce) package feta cheese, diced, divided

1 teaspoon minced fresh oregano, or to taste

Directions

Peel off a few strips of cucumber skin using a channel knife, creating a striped pattern. Cut cucumbers in half crosswise. Cut each half into quarters before cutting into 1/4- to 1/2-inch slices. Place into a colander; toss with some kosher salt and let sit for 10 to 15 minutes.

Meanwhile, cut cherry tomatoes in half. Rinse cucumbers; drain thoroughly for 10 to 15 minutes more.

While cucumbers are draining, slice onion thinly. Cut bell pepper into strips. Turn knife diagonally and cut strips into diamond-shaped pieces. Slice Kalamata and green olives.

Combine cucumbers, tomatoes, onion, bell pepper, olives, and 2 tablespoons oregano in a bowl. Season with salt, black pepper, and cayenne. Sprinkle in vinegar and toss thoroughly. Drizzle in olive oil. Add about 2/3 of the feta cheese and toss again. Cover with plastic wrap and refrigerate for 30 to 60 minutes.

Give the salad another mix. Taste and season as desired. Scatter remaining feta cheese on top and garnish with remaining oregano.

Chef's Notes:

If you need to make this the day before, I suggest making the dressing separately, and then mixing everything before the event. I think this should only be dressed about 30 to 60 minutes before service for maximum enjoyment, but that's just my approach, and some folks prefer an overnight marination.

Use 1/2 teaspoon dried oregano if you don't have the fresh kind.

Between 4 and 6 ounces of feta cheese work well here.

Nutrition Facts (per serving)

352 Calories

32g Fat

13g Carbs

6g Protein

Mediterranean Greek Salad

This is a great salad to take to a barbeque. All ingredients are approximate, so add more or less of any ingredient depending on your own taste.

Prep Time: 10 mins

Total Time: 10 mins

Servings: 8

Yield: 8 servings

Ingredients

3 cucumbers, seeded and sliced

1 ½ cups crumbled feta cheese

1 cup black olives, pitted and sliced

3 cups diced roma tomatoes

⅓ cup diced oil packed sun-dried tomatoes, drained, oil reserved

½ red onion, sliced

Directions

In a large salad bowl, toss together the cucumbers, feta cheese, olives, roma tomatoes, sun-dried tomatoes, 2 tablespoons reserved sun-dried tomato oil, and red onion. Chill until serving.

Nutrition Facts (per serving)

131 Calories 9g Fat 9g Carbs 6g Protein

Easy Greek Salad

This Greek cucumber salad with red onion, tomatoes, and feta cheese is a wonderful summer salad.

Prep Time: 15 mins

Total Time: 15 mins

Servings: 6

Ingredients

3 large ripe tomatoes, chopped

2 medium cucumbers, peeled and chopped

1 small red onion, chopped

¼ cup olive oil

4 teaspoons lemon juice

1 ½ teaspoons dried oregano

salt and pepper to taste

1 cup crumbled feta cheese

6 black Greek olives, pitted and sliced

Directions

Gather all ingredients.

Toss tomatoes, cucumbers, and red onion together in a shallow salad bowl.

Drizzle oil and lemon juice over top, then sprinkle with oregano, salt, and pepper.

Top with feta and olives. Enjoy!

Recipe Tip

You can use two green onions instead of a small red onion if desired.

Nutrition Facts (per serving)

187 Calories

16g Fat

8g Carbs

5g Protein

Lentil Rice and Veggie Bake

This delicious vegan lentil bake can be quickly thrown together from things you probably already have in the kitchen.

Prep Time: 15 mins

Cook Time: 1 hr

Total Time: 1 hr 15 mins

Servings: 6

Ingredients

½ cup uncooked long grain white rice

2 ½ cups water

1 cup red lentils

1 teaspoon vegetable oil

1 small onion, chopped

3 cloves garlic, minced

1 fresh tomato, chopped

⅓ cup chopped celery

⅓ cup chopped carrots

⅓ cup chopped zucchini

1 (8-ounce) can tomato sauce

1 teaspoon dried basil

1 teaspoon dried oregano

1 teaspoon ground cumin

salt and pepper, to taste

Directions

Place rice and 1 cup water in a pot and bring to a boil. Cover, reduce heat to low, and simmer 20 minutes. Place lentils in a pot with remaining 1 1/2 cups water, and bring to a boil. Cook 15 minutes, or until tender.

Preheat the oven to 350 degrees F (175 degrees C).

Heat oil in a skillet over medium heat, and stir in onion and garlic. Mix in tomato, celery, carrots, zucchini, and 1/2 the tomato sauce. Season with 1/2 the basil, 1/2 the oregano, 1/2 the cumin, salt, and pepper. Cook until vegetables are tender.

In a casserole dish, mix rice, lentils, and vegetables. Top with remaining tomato sauce and sprinkle with remaining basil, oregano, and cumin

Bake 30 minutes in the preheated oven, until bubbly.

Nutrition Facts (per serving)

187 Calories 2g Fat 35g Carbs 10g Protein

Delicious Lentil Loaf

I know nobody expects the words 'lentils' and 'delicious' in the same recipe title, but this lentil loaf is a hit with vegans, vegetarians and even meat-eaters! I've left the glaze open to your own tastes, you can use anything from barbeque sauce to your own mother's meatloaf glaze. Please add your glaze recipes into the comments!

Prep Time: 15 mins

Cook Time: 1 hr 25 mins

Additional Time: 10 mins

Total Time: 1 hr 50 mins

Servings: 6

Yield: 1 loaf

Ingredients

Lentil Loaf:

2 ½ cups water

1 cup brown lentils

⅓ cup water

3 tablespoons ground flax seed

2 tablespoons olive oil

1 onion, minced

1 cup minced fresh mushrooms

1 cup minced celery

2 large cloves garlic, minced

¾ cup quick-cooking oats

½ cup all-purpose flour

1 teaspoon dried basil

1 teaspoon ground black pepper

1 teaspoon salt

½ teaspoon onion powder

Glaze:

¼ cup ketchup

¼ cup brown sugar

2 tablespoons mustard

2 tablespoons smoky barbeque sauce

Directions

Combine 2 1/2 cups water and lentils in a saucepan; bring to a boil. Reduce heat, cover saucepan, and simmer until all the liquid is absorbed and lentils are tender, 20 to 30 minutes.

Mix 1/3 cup water and ground flax seed together in a bowl; set aside until thickened, at least 10 minutes.

Heat olive oil in a large pot over medium heat; cook and stir onion, mushrooms, celery, and garlic until softened and liquid from mushrooms has evaporated, 5 to 10 minutes.

Preheat oven to 350 degrees F (175 degrees C). Grease a loaf pan.

Transfer cooked lentils to a food processor and pulse until about 75 percent of lentils are mashed. Mix onion-mushroom mixture, flax seed-water mixture, oats, flour, basil, black pepper, salt, and onion powder into lentils until well combined. Press lentil mixture into the prepared loaf pan.

Combine ketchup, brown sugar, mustard, and barbeque sauce in a saucepan over medium-low heat; cook and stir until glaze is smooth and brown sugar is dissolved, about 5 minutes. Remove saucepan from heat.

Bake loaf in the preheated oven for 35 minutes. Spread 1/4 cup glaze over lentil loaf; continue baking until cooked through, 10 to 15 minutes more. Serve lentil loaf with remaining glaze on the side.

Recipe Tips

You can substitute vegetable stock for the water, dried oregano for the dried basil, and dehydrated onion for the onion powder.

If you don't have a food processor, you can mash the lentils with a fork instead.

Nutrition Facts (per serving)

318 Calories 8g Fat 51g Carbs 13g Protein

Lentil Loaf

This vegetarian staple features a crunchy bread crumb topping. Make it the centerpiece of your meal, and serve with a savory vegetarian gravy, mashed potatoes, and English peas.

Prep Time: 45 mins

Cook Time: 50 mins

Total Time: 1 hr 35 mins

Servings: 6

Yield: 6 servings

Ingredients

1 ⅛ cups green lentils

2 ¼ cups water

6 slices white bread, torn into small pieces

2 eggs

1 cup vegetable broth

2 tablespoons tomato paste

½ teaspoon dried basil

¼ teaspoon garlic powder

½ teaspoon ground black pepper

1 teaspoon dried parsley

1 tablespoon olive oil

½ packet dry vegetable soup mix

⅓ cup dried bread crumbs

Directions

Combine lentils and water in a small saucepan. Bring to a boil. Reduce heat, and simmer until tender, about 40 minutes.

Preheat oven to 400 degrees F (205 degrees C). Grease a 9x5 inch loaf pan.

In a large bowl, mix together 2 cups cooked lentils, bread, eggs, broth, tomato paste, basil, garlic powder, black pepper, parsley, olive oil, and dry soup mix. Spread into prepared pan.

Bake for 40 minutes. Sprinkle top with dry bread crumbs, and continue baking another 10 minutes. Let sit for 10 minutes before serving.

Nutrition Facts (per serving)

272 Calories 6g Fat 41g Carbs 15g Protein

My mom came up with this recipe for cheesy lentils when I was a teenage vegetarian. It's still one of my favorite dishes to this day, and my meat-loving husband loves it too!

Prep Time: 25 mins

Cook Time: 1 hr 15 mins

Total Time: 1 hr 40 mins

Servings: 6

Ingredients

2 cups water

1 ⅔ cups dry lentils

1 (14.5 ounce) can stewed tomatoes

2 large onions, chopped

3 cloves garlic, minced

2 teaspoons salt

¼ teaspoon pepper

¼ teaspoon dried marjoram

¼ teaspoon dried sage

¼ teaspoon dried thyme

1 large bay leaf

2 large carrots, cut into 1/2 inch pieces

1 stalk celery, chopped

1 medium green bell pepper, chopped

1 ½ cups shredded sharp Cheddar cheese

Directions

Preheat the oven to 375 degrees F (190 degrees C).

Mix water, lentils, stewed tomatoes, onions, garlic, salt, pepper, marjoram, sage, thyme, and bay leaf together in a 3-quart casserole dish.

Bake, uncovered, in the preheated oven for 30 minutes.

Stir in carrots and celery; cover and continue to bake until lentils and vegetables are tender, about 40 minutes.

Stir in bell pepper, then sprinkle Cheddar over top. Bake, uncovered, until cheese has melted, about 5 more minutes. Remove bay leaf before serving.

Nutrition Facts (per serving)

383 Calories 12g Fat 45g Carbs 24g Protein

Unlike most of America's other favorite fast foods, falafel is rarely attempted at home, which is a shame, since it's very simple to do, and even a relative novice like me can get some very decent results. One word of warning: you do need to know you're going to have a craving for this a full day before you actually want to eat it.

Prep Time: 20 mins

Cook Time: 10 mins

Additional Time: 12 hrs

Total Time: 12 hrs 30 mins

Servings: 6

Yield: 6 servings

Ingredients

1 cup dry garbanzo beans

½ yellow onion, diced

½ cup chopped fresh flat-leaf parsley

4 cloves minced garlic

1 tablespoon all-purpose flour, or more as needed

2 teaspoons lemon juice

1 ½ teaspoons salt, or to taste

1 teaspoon ground cumin

½ teaspoon ground coriander

¼ teaspoon baking soda

⅛ teaspoon cayenne pepper

oil for frying

Directions

Place garbanzo beans into a large container and cover with several inches of cool water; let stand 12 to 24 hours. Drain.

Blend garbanzo beans, onion, parsley, garlic, flour, lemon juice, salt, cumin, coriander, baking soda, and cayenne pepper together in a food processor, scraping down the sides of the bowl as necessary, until mixture is finely ground and holds together when pressed. Transfer garbanzo mixture to a bowl, cover with plastic wrap, and refrigerate until flavors blend, 1 to 2 hours.

Heat oil in a deep-fryer or large saucepan to 350 degrees F (175 degrees C).

Divide dough into 12 portions and roll each with moistened hands into a ball.

Working in batches, cook falafel balls in hot oil until browned and crispy, about 5 minutes. Transfer to a wire rack to drain.

Nutrition Facts (per serving)

271 Calories 17g Fat 24g Carbs 7g Protein

Baked Falafel

An easy, yummy way to make falafel. Serve with pita bread and your favorite tzatziki.

Prep Time: 20 mins

Cook Time: 20 mins

Additional Time:15 mins

Total Time: 55 mins

Servings: 2

Yield: 4 patties

Ingredients

¼ cup chopped onion

1 (15 ounce) can garbanzo beans, rinsed and drained

¼ cup chopped fresh parsley

3 cloves garlic, minced

1 teaspoon ground cumin

¼ teaspoon ground coriander

¼ teaspoon salt

¼ teaspoon baking soda

1 tablespoon all-purpose flour

1 egg, beaten

2 teaspoons olive oil

Directions

Wrap onion in cheese cloth and squeeze out as much moisture as possible. Set aside. Place garbanzo beans, parsley, garlic, cumin, coriander, salt, and baking soda in a food processor. Process until the mixture is coarsely pureed. Mix garbanzo bean mixture and onion together in a bowl. Stir in the flour and egg. Shape mixture into four large patties and let stand for 15 minutes.

Preheat an oven to 400 degrees F (200 degrees C).

Heat olive oil in a large, oven-safe skillet over medium-high heat. Place the patties in the skillet; cook until golden brown, about 3 minutes on each side.

Transfer skillet to the preheated oven and bake until heated through, about 10 minutes.

Nutrition Facts (per serving)

281 Calories 9g Fat 39g Carbs 11g Protein

Three Bean Salad

This tasty three bean salad is great for buffets, summer picnics, and cookouts. It's easy to make but tastes best when chilled for at least 12 hours. It keeps well and serves a lot of people.

Prep Time: 15 mins

Additional Time: 12 hrs

Total Time: 12 hrs 15 mins

Servings: 16

Ingredients

1 (15 ounce) can green beans

1 pound wax beans

1 (15 ounce) can kidney beans, drained and rinsed

1 onion, sliced into thin rings

¾ cup white sugar, or to taste

⅔ cup distilled white vinegar

⅓ cup vegetable oil

½ teaspoon salt

½ teaspoon ground black pepper

½ teaspoon celery seed

Directions

Gather all ingredients.

Mix together green beans, wax beans, kidney beans, onion, sugar, vinegar, vegetable oil, salt, pepper, and celery seed. Chill in refrigerator for at least 12 hours.

Enjoy!

Nutrition Facts (per serving)

112 Calories 5g Fat 16g Carbs 2g Protein

Easy Three Bean Salad

We like to make this tasty three-bean salad to serve with a variety of other salads when we prepare a buffet. It's easy to make, keeps well, and serves a lot of people! This salad is also great for summer picnics and cookouts.

Prep Time: 15 mins

Additional Time: 12 hrs

Total Time: 12 hrs 15 mins

Servings: 16

Ingredients

1 (15-ounce) can green beans, drained

1 (14.5-ounce) can yellow wax beans, drained

1 (15-ounce) can kidney beans, drained and rinsed

1 onion, sliced into thin rings

¾ cup white sugar

⅔ cup distilled white vinegar

⅓ cup vegetable oil

½ teaspoon salt

½ teaspoon ground black pepper

½ teaspoon celery seed

Directions

Mix green beans, wax beans, kidney beans, onion, sugar, vinegar, vegetable oil, salt, pepper, and celery seed together in a large salad bowl; cover and chill in the refrigerator for at least 12 hours.

Nutrition Facts (per serving)

112 Calories 5g Fat 16g Carbs 2g Protein

This recipe was given to me by a vegan friend I had in college. It is the best bean salad I have ever tasted, and I love it because you can experiment with the ingredients and still have a mouth-watering side dish. I hope you like it!

Prep Time: 15 mins

Additional Time: 2 hrs

Total Time: 2 hrs 15 mins

Servings: 8

Yield: 8 servings

Ingredients

1 (15 ounce) can garbanzo beans (chickpeas), drained and rinsed

1 (15 ounce) can kidney beans, drained and rinsed

1 (15 ounce) can green beans, drained and rinsed

4 green onions, chopped

1 stalk celery, sliced

½ cup cider vinegar

¼ cup vegetable oil

1 tablespoon honey

½ teaspoon ground dry mustard

¼ teaspoon garlic powder

¼ teaspoon ground black pepper

¼ teaspoon onion powder (Optional)

¼ teaspoon ground cayenne pepper (Optional)

Directions

In a bowl, gently mix the garbanzo beans, kidney beans, green beans, green onions, and celery. In a separate bowl, whisk together the vinegar, oil, honey, mustard, garlic powder, black pepper, onion powder, and cayenne pepper. Pour dressing over the salad, and toss gently to coat. Cover, refrigerate at least 2 hours, and gently toss before serving.

Nutrition Facts (per serving)

170Calories 8g Fat 21g Carbs 5g Protein

Spicy Black Bean Salad
Great with tortilla chips. Serve chilled.

Prep Time: 15 mins

Additional Time: 1 hr

Total Time: 1 hr 15 mins

Servings: 10

Yield: 10 servings

Ingredients

2 (15 ounce) cans black beans, drained and rinsed

1 (15.25 ounce) can whole kernel corn, drained

1 red onion, diced

¾ cup salsa, or as desired

½ cup olive oil

½ cup chopped fresh cilantro

3 cloves garlic, minced

2 tablespoons lemon juice

1 tablespoon red wine vinegar

1 ½ teaspoons ground cumin

1 teaspoon salt

¼ teaspoon ground black pepper

Directions

Mix black beans, corn, red onion, salsa, olive oil, cilantro, garlic, lemon juice, vinegar, cumin, salt, and black pepper in a large bowl. Cover and refrigerate at least 1 hour to 2 days. Serve chilled.

Nutrition Facts (per serving)

221 Calories 12g Fat 25g Carbs 7g Protein

Panzanella Salad

Panzanella is an Italian bread, tomato, and red onion salad that is packed with flavor and different textures. I love to add mozzarella cheese and olives.

Prep Time: 30 mins

Cook Time: 20 mins

Total Time: 50 mins

Servings: 8

Ingredients

6 cups day old Italian bread, torn into bite-size pieces

⅓ cup olive oil

salt and pepper to taste

3 cloves garlic, minced

¼ cup olive oil

2 tablespoons balsamic vinegar

4 medium ripe tomatoes, cut into wedges

¾ cup sliced red onion

10 basil leaves, shredded

½ cup pitted and halved green olives

1 cup fresh mozzarella, cut into bite-size pieces

Directions

Preheat the oven to 400 degrees F (200 degrees C).

Toss bread with 1/3 cup olive oil, salt, pepper, and garlic in a large bowl; arrange on a baking sheet and toast in the preheated oven until golden, about 5 to 10 minutes. Transfer bread back into the bowl and set aside to cool slightly.

Whisk 1/4 cup of olive oil and balsamic vinegar together in a small bowl; set aside.

Add tomatoes, onion, basil, olives, and mozzarella cheese into the bowl with bread; toss with vinaigrette and let stand for 20 minutes before serving.

Nutrition Facts (per serving)

335 Calories 24g Fat 22g Carbs 9g Protein

Grilled Panzanella Salad with Peaches and Fennel

This is a hearty but bright salad using the colors and flavors of the summer season from Lindsey S. Love of Dolly and Oatmeal. The bread is rubbed with garlic and brushed with olive oil then grilled until toasty and crunchy. The peaches are also grilled until warm and slightly caramelized, and the fennel is shaved thin, giving the salad brightness and crunch.

Prep Time: 30 mins

Cook Time: 15 mins

Additional Time: 10 mins

Total Time: 55 mins

Servings: 4

Yield: 4 servings

Ingredients

1 large shallot, sliced thin

2 tablespoons white wine vinegar

1 teaspoon maple syrup (or sweetener of choice)

½ teaspoon fine sea salt and fresh pepper

6 tablespoons extra-virgin olive oil, divided

1 clove garlic

4 slices hearty bread

2 peaches, sliced into wedges

2 cups baby arugula

1 cup torn basil leaves

1 large fennel bulb, halved, cored and thinly shaved
on a mandoline

Reynolds Wrap® Non Stick Aluminum Foil

Directions

Cut a large piece of Reynolds Wrap® Non Stick Aluminum Foil and firmly fit it over the grill grate. Heat the grill to medium heat.

While the grill is heating, make the dressing. To a shallow bowl, add the shallot, vinegar, maple syrup, and a couple pinches of salt and pepper to taste. Let the mixture sit until the shallots are tender, about 10 minutes. Add 4 tablespoons of the oil and whisk until the dressing is mixed and blended. Set aside.

Cut the garlic clove in half. Gently rub both sides of each slice of bread with the cut side of the garlic. Using 1 tablespoon of oil, lightly brush each side of the bread.

Place the bread on the hot grill and cook until toasted and firm, about 7 to 10 minutes. Remove the bread and let cool.

Brush the peaches with the remaining tablespoon of oil and sprinkle with a couple pinches of salt. Place the peaches on the foil-covered grill and cook until lightly browned but firm, about 4 to 5 minutes. Remove from heat and set aside.

In a large serving bowl, toss together the arugula and basil. Tear the bread into large chunks and add to the bowl. Add the peaches and fennel. Mix in the dressing and give everything a thorough toss.

Reynolds Kitchens Tip

Use Reynolds Wrap(R) Non-Stick Foil to prevent items like vegetables, fruit or smaller pieces of food from falling between the grill grates.

Nutrition Facts (per serving)

289 Calories 21g Fat 22g Carbs 3g Protein

Panzanella Salad with Bison Flank Steak

Flavorful grilled bison flank steak is sliced thinly across the grain for maximum tenderness and served with an Italian-inspired toasted bread salad with tomatoes, fresh mozzarella cheese, and basil leaves.

Prep Time: 40 mins

Cook Time: 8 mins

Total Time: 48 mins

Servings: 6

Yield: 6 servings

Ingredients

4 ounces dried French bread, torn into bite-size pieces

2 tablespoons olive oil

1 cup chopped fresh mozzarella cheese

2 cups coarsely chopped seeded red or yellow tomatoes

1 cup seeded chopped cucumber

1 cup thinly sliced red onion

⅓ cup chopped fresh basil

3 tablespoons white wine vinegar

3 tablespoons olive oil

3 cloves garlic, minced

½ teaspoon salt

¼ teaspoon black pepper

Grilled Bison Flank Steak:

1 pound bison flank steak

½ teaspoon salt

⅛ teaspoon black pepper

Directions

Preheat oven to 450 degrees F. Place bread pieces in a shallow baking pan. Drizzle with the 2 tablespoons oil; toss gently to coat. Bake for 5 minutes or until toasted, stirring once or twice. Cool slightly; transfer to a very large bowl.

Combine mozzarella cheese, tomatoes, cucumber, onion, and basil in a large bowl; set aside.

For dressing, whisk together vinegar, the 3 tablespoons oil, the garlic, the 1/2 teaspoon salt, and the 1/4 teaspoon pepper in a small bowl. Pour dressing over the tomato mixture; toss to coat. Spoon the tomato mixture over the bread; toss to coat. Let stand for 15 minutes to allow the flavors to blend. Serve with Grilled Bison Flank Steak.

Grilled Bison Flank Steak: Sprinkle bison flank steak with the 1 teaspoon salt and the 1/4 teaspoon pepper. For gas or charcoal grill, place steak on the rack of an uncovered grill directly over medium-high heat. Grill for 8 to 10 minutes or until desired doneness. Cover bison flank steak with foil and let stand for 5 minutes. Thinly slice steak across the grain.

Tips

Note: Recipe developed and tested by the Better Homes and Gardens(R) Test Kitchen using High Plains Bison products.

Nutrition Facts (per serving)

304 Calories 17g Fat 17g Carbs 20g Protein

Italy's famous bread salad is usually associated with Tuscany, but my husband's father emigrated from Sicily, so I made up this version of bread salad using the flavors of Sicilian cuisine.

Prep Time: 40 mins

Cook Time: 12 mins

Additional Time: 40 mins

Total Time: 1 hr 32 mins

Servings: 10

Yield: 10 servings

Ingredients

8 ounces country style white bread, cut into 1 inch cubes

3 tablespoons garlic flavored olive oil

½ teaspoon coarse salt

1 (15 ounce) can garbanzo beans, rinsed and drained

2 cups red or yellow teardrop tomatoes, halved

⅓ cup chopped green bell pepper

⅓ cup chopped red bell pepper

1 small red onion, cut into 3/4 inch slices

10 kalamata olives, pitted and halved

⅓ cup basil pesto

¼ cup balsamic vinegar

1 tablespoon minced fresh rosemary

¼ teaspoon black pepper

4 ounces crumbled goat cheese

1 head green or red leaf lettuce

¼ cup toasted pine nuts

Directions

Preheat oven to 350 degrees F (175 degrees C).

Toss the bread cubes with the olive oil to evenly coat. Sprinkle with salt, and toss again. Spread the cubed bread evenly over a baking sheet, and bake in the preheated oven until golden brown, about 12 minutes. Remove from oven and allow to cool completely.

Toss together the garbanzo beans, tomatoes, peppers, onion, and kalamata olives in a large bowl. In a separate bowl, whisk together the pesto, balsamic vinegar, rosemary, and pepper. Toss the tomatoes with the pesto mixture, and let stand at room temperature for 30 minutes to 1 hour.

To serve, toss the toasted bread cubes and goat cheese with the tomato mixture. Line a serving platter with a few lettuce leaves. Shred the remaining lettuce, and mound in the center of the platter. Spoon the bread mixture over the lettuce, and sprinkle with toasted pine nuts.

Nutrition Facts (per serving)

264 Calories 15g Fat 25g Carbs 9g Protein

I made this for my make-ahead cooking group "The Make-Ahead Mamas'" holiday soup swap. The wonderful traditional Moroccan cinnamon-spice combination is lovely with the ground lamb and sweet potatoes, and the chopped apricots or cranberries add a surprising tart sweetness with every few bites. Whenever I make this recipe, I make a double (or triple!) batch and freeze a few portions.

Prep Time: 30 mins

Cook Time: 30 mins

Additional Time:2 hrs

Total Time: 3 hrs

Servings: 8

Yield: 8 servings

Ingredients

1 pound ground lamb

1 teaspoon ground cinnamon

1 teaspoon ground cumin

1 teaspoon kosher salt

½ teaspoon ground ginger

¼ teaspoon ground cloves

¼ teaspoon ground nutmeg

¼ teaspoon ground turmeric

⅛ teaspoon curry powder

1 tablespoon butter

1 sweet onion, chopped

2 (10.5 ounce) cans beef consomme

1 (14.5 ounce) can diced tomatoes with juice

1 (14 ounce) can organic beef broth

1 (14 ounce) can organic chicken broth

1 tablespoon honey

3 large carrots, halved lengthwise and thinly sliced

2 sweet potatoes, peeled and diced

1 (15 ounce) can garbanzo beans, rinsed and drained

1 cup lentils, rinsed and drained

½ cup chopped dried apricots (Optional)

⅛ teaspoon cayenne pepper, or to taste (Optional)

1 pinch ground black pepper to taste

Directions

Mix ground lamb, cinnamon, cumin, salt, ginger, cloves, nutmeg, turmeric, and curry powder together in a bowl. Cover and put in the refrigerator for 2 hours to overnight.

Melt butter in a soup pot over medium-high heat; stir in onion. Cook, stirring frequently, until the onion has softened and turned translucent, 5 to 10 minutes. Reduce heat to medium and add spiced lamb mixture. Cook and stir until browned and crumbly, 5 to 7 minutes.

Add consomme, diced tomatoes, beef broth, chicken broth, and honey. Stir in carrots, sweet potatoes, garbanzo beans, lentils, apricots, cayenne pepper, and black pepper.

Bring soup just to a boil over medium-high heat, then reduce heat to low, and simmer until lentils and vegetables are tender, 15 to 20 minutes.

Cook's Notes:

Barley can be used in place of lentils, and dried cranberries can be used in place of apricots.

To make this soup ahead, I suggest not cooking the soup fully until just before serving it, so that the vegetables stay firm while frozen. Follow steps 1 to 3, then transfer soup to a freezer-safe container. Place in the refrigerator for up to 3 days, or freeze. When ready to eat, if refrigerated, simply transfer to a pot and follow step 4. If frozen, thaw in the the refrigerator for 24 to 48 hours, pour into a soup pot, and follow step 4.

Nutrition Facts (per serving)

382 Calories 10g Fat 49g Carbs 24g Protein

Conclusion

Many people with fibromyalgia find certain foods can trigger a flare-up. Sugar, gluten, dairy, and fried or processed foods can lead to symptoms like widespread muscle pain (myalgia) and fatigue.

The connection between the foods you eat and fibromyalgia pain is not well understood. Some evidence suggests food allergies or intolerances may be to blame. Other research links fibromyalgia symptoms to nutritional deficiencies, such as iron, vitamin D, and B-complex vitamins.

There is no one-size-fits-all fibromyalgia diet plan. The overall goal is to avoid foods that increase neuron excitability that triggers fibromyalgia symptoms. At the same time, you want to add anti-inflammatory foods that help prevent fibromyalgia flares.

A fibromyalgia diet should be approached strategically and rationally: Making sudden or extreme changes—even healthy ones—can trigger a fibromyalgia flare.

Some food sensitivities are easier to deal with than others. If you find you're sensitive to gluten, for instance, you may benefit from speaking with a dietitian or nutritionist to learn about the many foods you'll need to avoid and how to replace lost nutrients with "safe" foods.

Whatever diet plan you embark on, keep to a regular schedule of at least three meals per day unless your healthcare provider tells you otherwise. Skipping meals can lead to overeating, which not only causes stomach upset and fatigue but induces inflammation.

If you feel hungry between meals, keep to healthy snacks like fruits, vegetables, and hummus (100% natural).